P³

the power of**THREE**

You've followed all the weight loss rules.
You've started working out, you've bought the weight loss
supplements, meal prepped your food, and...
it should be working by now, but it's not!
You are frustrated and exhausted to no end! It doesn't seem fair!
If you are craving a solution to put you in control of your weight...
then you need to start here... with the POWER OF 3

Jennifer H. Armstrong

the POWER of 3

What's the deal with the always flip-flopping nutritional advice in the media? Turn on the local news and every day there's new information on what's REALLY bad for you. Is it calories? Sugar? Fat? Carbs? The supplement aisle — heck, whole chains of STORES are full of vitamins and other stuff, and most of it is not FDA-approved. We all have tried (I tend to go with how the logo looks, mid-price point, and frankly, the color of the bottle). And then there are the "movements:" the "farm to table" movement, the "whole foods" movement, the "eat only a third of your plate at a restaurant" movement and let's not even get into what "organic" means anymore. The list goes on and on until the anxiety of choice leads you to a small conniption fit in aisle 12.

The Secret Revealed? Atkins, Weight Watchers, Jenny Craig, Even Subway, for goodness' sake! Everyone and every company seems to have the "secret" to eating right and losing weight. There are plenty of magazines you can subscribe to, each basically recycling the same tips. The 20 Easy Ways To... self-help books seem to be a vibrant market. You purchase one with the hope THIS will be the key to your weight loss. But then, on day one, you flip

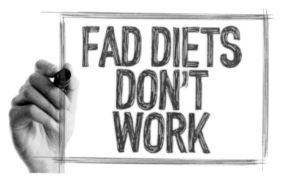

through the first chapter, skip the first "worksheet" and "journal" pages at the end, and swear you'll start the regimen tomorrow. Before long, you file it next to the cookbooks, that you've never used either.

You'll probably be relieved to hear me say that diets don't work... none of them do!!

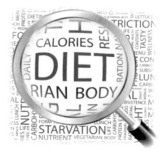

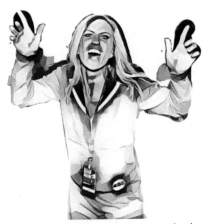

Even though you've been blaming yourself this entire time, somewhere in the back of your mind you knew it was the diet that was failing you. The truth is that calorie restriction doesn't work long-term. Cutting out all carbs does not work long term. Carb cycling does not work, and fasting does not work for a long time. These lead to the endless cycle of weight loss and weight gain; the see-saw you've been on your whole life! What about the exercise? You're led to believe that exercise is the all-important factor, controlling somewhere around 80% of your body composition. That's why the gym industry has completely exploded in popularity with people trying to sculpt the body they've always wanted. The truth is, exercise isn't all that important either. With regard for the big picture, exercise controls about 20% of your body composition. It's not because you're not eating six small meals a day, it's not because you're too lazy to slave away at a boot camp five days a week, it's not because you don't own a treadmill, it's not because you eat dinner after 6pm; it's not because of any of that nonsense. So why are so many people overweight?....in my truths ... it can be one of two reasons... 1. You are Insulin resistant, or 2. Your metabolism is out of whack. You're metabolically broken and/or insulin resistant NOT because of how much you eat and how little you exercise, but simply because of what you eat. Your body is at war with what you're feeding it. Your hormones are out of whack, causing you to store more fat and you've done so much damage that your fat cells have lost the ability to release the fat you've stored. With the proper nutrition, rest, recovery and underlying unhealthy issues of how you perceive your self-worth!!!

The power of 3 is a lifestyle change, not a diet! It includes proper foods, proper rest, adequate recovery time along with sufficient exercise and daily affirmations that your improving your self image!

You need balance and nutrition, fitness and stability in your personal life! You need consistency in all of these areas as well! Diets, for the most part are tedious temporary fixes. Rule number one - if you cannot sustain it for a lifetime, never start it to begin with! The power of three creates a lifetime of positive changes!

ON YOUR REST DAY

a day you do nothing but chill! The Value of Rest. It is rest that makes you stronger, because it is rest that allows the muscles you have broken down to heal and recover. It is the rest that allows you to recover so you can be strong, and thereby handle the increased weight, and increased number of sets and reps needed to gain further. So on your rest days you are going to feed your body the healthy healing foods it needs to rebuild.

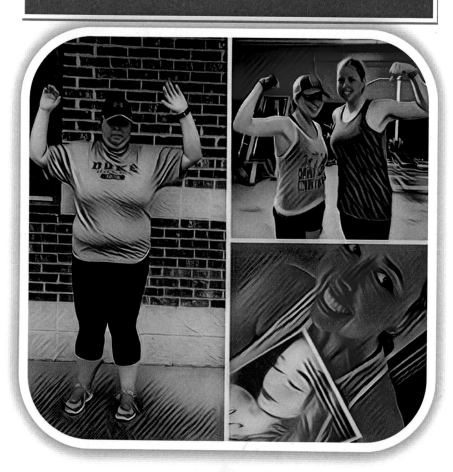

meal plan
your 3 recovery days

Breakfast

phat coffee - coffee brewed
Ubrew- 1 teaspoon of MCT oil- 1 tablespoon of coconut oil
Drink -I teaspoon of Braggs Apple Cider Vinegar
with 16oz of water with lemon

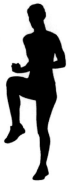

Lunch

3 oz of shrimp or crab meat or tuna
On a bed of :
2 cups of spinach or spring mix
¼ cup blackberries
¼ cup of onions
¼ cup celery chopped
1 oz goat cheese
Drizzle with EVOO and a teaspoon of Braggs Apple Cider Vinegar
3 cups of water with lemon

Dinner

3 oz of a low sugar wine- optional
3 oz steak / beef or salmon or Mahi Mahi
(You can chop up 1 slice of bacon
to top protein with as well) cooked and topped
with EVOO and 1 oz goat cheese
1 cup broccoli chopped and sautéed in EVOO
1 cup mushroom chopped and sautéed in EVOO
20 macadamia nuts

> No snacks
> during the day
> 1 gallon of water
> 1 ZipFizz
> pre workout

recovery is vital to

Repair muscle and tissue.
Remove waste products and reduce inflammation….
this is why we have increased fiber on these days

Replenish energy stores nutrients necessary for cellular activity.
Restore the central nervous system , which, in simple terms,
is repairing the connection between the brain and body- keep moving…

approved swap foods list

FATS	FIBERS	PROTEINS	BEVERAGES
Extra Virgin Olive Oil	Spinach	Eggs	3oz Low Sugar Wine
Avocado Oil	Kale	Salmon	Unsweetened Tea
MCT Oil	Broccoli	Mackerel	Water
Coconut Oil	Cabbage	Tuna	Herbal Tea
Macadamia Nuts	Cauliflower	Crab	San Pellegrino
Walnuts	Celery	Shrimp	Zip Fizz
Pecans	Cucumber	Oysters	
Olives	Tomato	Sardines	
Brie	Garlic	Snapper	
Goat Cheese	Bell Peppers	Anchovies	
Avocados	Mustard Greens	Flounder	
	Peppers	Mahi Mahi	
	Egg Plant	Bacon	
	Blueberries	Unglazed Ham	
	Raspberries	Chicken	
	Spring Mix Romain	Beef	
	Mushrooms		
	Bok Choy		
	Onions		
	Shallots		
	Radishes		

foods & ingredients to avoid

Added sugar: Soda, candy, ice cream, table sugar and many others.
Refined grains: White bread, pasta made with refined wheat, etc.
Trans fats: found in margarine and various processed foods.
Refined Oils: soybean oil, canola oil, cottonseed oil and others.
Processed meat: processed sausages, hot dogs, etc.
Highly processed foods: Everything labeled "low-fat" or "diet"
or looks like it was made in a factory.

You MUST read the labels

if you want to avoid these unhealthy ingredients.

supplements

Potassium at each meal • Magnesium at bedtime
Digestive enzymes at each meal

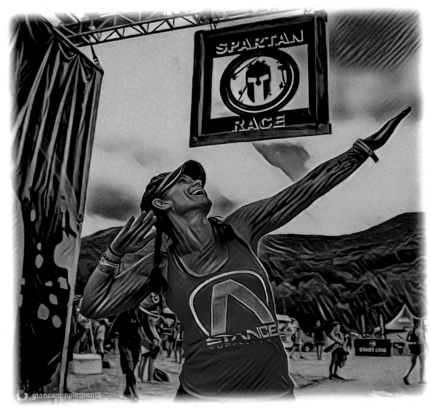

your training plan

3

Intense workouts per week

Recovery days (see list below)

One day of rest - unplug & reset!

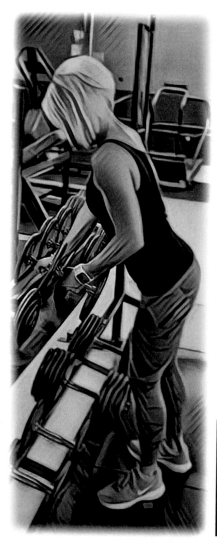

recovery

choose 3 per week:

- Yoga
- Deep stretches
- Hot Epsom salt bath
- Massage therapy
- Manicure or pedicure
- Sex
- Brisk walk
- Reading
- Power nap
- If running is your "Therapy" you can add it as well
- Herbal teas...

Unplug from any social media, TV, extra or extended work hours

1 cheat meal of your choice
1 time per month
you can have anything you
want, in one sitting

your training plan
exercise

- Warm up 5 minute- light walk on the treadmill at a 7% incline at 2.5 speed

3 rounds of 10 reps with no rest
MHR 75%

- Kettlebell swings
- Box jumps
- Squat jumps

Rest 60 seconds

3 rounds of 10 reps with no rest

- Medicine ball jumping jacks
- Mtn. climbers
- Burpees

Rest 60 seconds

5 rounds of 8 to 10 reps with moderate weight

- Military press with dumbbells
- Front raise to over head with a bar
- Arnold press with a static hold for 5 seconds

5 rounds of 10 reps

- Hammer front raises
- Upright rows with a bar
- Push press with dumbbells
- 5 rounds of 10 reps
- Seated lateral raises
- Shoulder shrugs
- Front to lateral raises

*Be sure to log the amount of weight and reps you were able to complete.

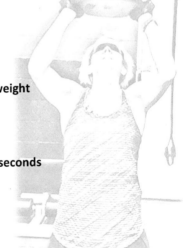

your training plan
exercise

- Warm up for 5 minutes on the Stair-mill

- 10 minute Treadmill sprints

- Set your timer for 30 seconds, you will jog 30 seconds and sprint 30 seconds MHR 85%

5 rounds-do not set the bar down- keep moving-lighter weight

- 2 front squats

- 2 push press

- 2 back squats

- 10 reverse lunges with bar on your back

3 rounds of 10

- Burpee of the bar

- Squat jumps

- Good Morning with a calf raise with a bar

3 rounds of 10 (heavy weights)

- Back squat

- Dumbbell plié squat

- Body weight squats

DON'T YOU DARE QUIT!

your training plan
exercise

5 minute warm up on the treadmill.....steady walk, no incline

ONE BIG REP

You will set your timer for 60 minutes, completing each exercise-moving on to the next one without rest

Do this circuit AMRAP (as many times as possible within that 60 minutes) MHR 85%

- 10 chest press on a bench with dumbbells
- 10 dips on bench
- 10 wide pushups
- 10 tricep extensions with dumbbell
- 10 chest press on the bench with dumbbells
- 10 burpees
- 10 skull crushers
- 10 chest flies on the bench with dumbbells
- 10 wide pushups
- 10 dips on the bench
- 10 tricep extensions with a dumbbells
- 10 burpees
- 10 chest press on the bench with dumbbells
- 10 skull crushers with dumbbell
- Be sure to log the number of rounds and amount of weight you were able to complete

Be your own superhero

your training plan
exercise

Warm up on the treadmill with a
5 minute brisk walk -MHR 70%

4 rounds of 12 reps

Wide grip lat pull down

Seated row

One arm dumbbell row (each arm)

3 rounds of 10 reps

Hammer curls

Renegade rows

Plank to failure

4 rounds of 12 reps

Bent over dumbbell fly

Wide curls with bar

Narrow pull ups

3 rounds of 10 reps

Underhanded row with a bar

Chin ups and Wide pull ups

I'm not telling you it is
going to be easy,
I'm telling you
it's going to be worth it.

your training plan
exercise

Warm up 10 minutes on the stair-mill

Treadmill sprints for 10 minutes, set your timer for 60/30- you will jog for 60 seconds and sprint hard for 30 seconds. MHR 85%

5 rounds of 7 reps (heavy)

Back squats

100 meter run

3 rounds of 10 reps

1 legged deadlift - right leg-right hand with a kettlebell

1 legged deadlift- left hand -right leg with a kettlebell

Goblet squat

4 rounds of 12 reps

Leg press- increase weight after each set of 12

Calve raises on the leg press

3 rounds of 10- reps

Leg extensions (hold and squeeze at the top) you will do a set of unilateral and bi-lateral)

*both legs for a set-left leg for a set-right leg for a set

2 rounds of 25 reps

Hip thruster

Bulgarian split lunges

i can and i will.
watch me.

your training plan
exercise weeks 5 - 12

20 minute Treadmill 80% MHR

Time Incline Speed

0-5:00 minutes 0-2% 3.5-4 mph

5-6:00 minutes 5% 5-6 mph

6-7:00 minutes 2% 4 mph

7-9:00 minutes 10% 5-6 mph

9-10:00 minutes 15% 3 mph

10-11:00 minutes 5 % 4 mph

11-15:00 minutes 10% 5-6 mph

15-16:00 minutes 2% 3.5 mph

16-20:00 15% 4 mph

YOU DID NOT WAKE UP TODAY TO BE MEDIOCRE

4 rounds of 10 (in between each set your active rest with be preformed)
Active rest 20 plank shoulder taps

Ex: 10 shoulder press + 20 plank shoulder taps 4 rounds
Follow the same format on the following exercises

4 rounds of 10 reps + 20 active rest:

Shoulder press + plank shoulder taps

Rest 60 seconds

4 rounds of 10 reps + 20 active rest

Alternating dumbbell shoulder press + shoulder push ups

Rest 60 seconds

4 rounds of 10 reps + 20 active rest

Weighted bar standing calve raises + squat jumps

Rest 60 seconds

4 rounds of 10 reps + 20 active rest

One arm upright row with smith machine + box jumps

Rest 60 seconds

4 rounds of 10 reps + 20 active rest

Weighted squats + Mt. climbers

Rest 60 seconds

3 rounds of 10 + 10 active rest

Arnold press + burpees

the MAKEOVER mindset

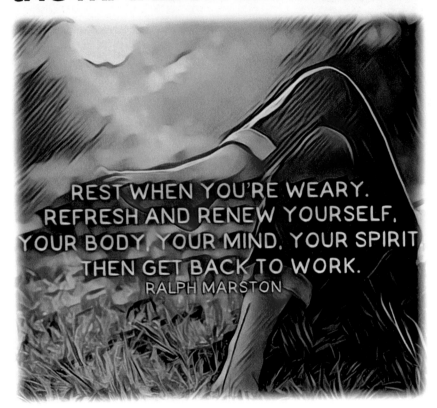

REST WHEN YOU'RE WEARY.
REFRESH AND RENEW YOURSELF,
YOUR BODY, YOUR MIND, YOUR SPIRIT,
THEN GET BACK TO WORK.
RALPH MARSTON

Each day journal the water / foods you consume, the training /recovery and rest you've completed. Document 3 areas you have improved in your life & 3 areas you need to make changes to.

Be real and honest! Self-Awareness is having a clear perception of your personality, including strengths, weaknesses, thoughts, beliefs, motivation, and emotions. Self-Awareness allows you to understand other people, how they perceive you, your attitude and your responses to them in the a positive way. Being real and aware will allow you to get rid of the *Emotional Drama* in your life! It will allow you to Stop Emotional Reactions, Change Core Beliefs, Quiet the Criticizing Voices in Your Head, and help Develop Communication and Respect in your Relationships.

Create Love and Happiness in Your Life! Its time you start to see your own value and find your inner strength!!

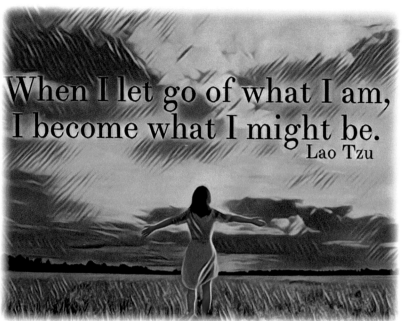

When I let go of what I am,
I become what I might be.
Lao Tzu

3 Things I need to change about my eating habits

cut out the sugar

portion control

less bread/snacking

✓ Things I need to add to my daily routine

quiet time (early)

reflection time (late)

✓ Things I need to start telling myself

I CAN do it!

I will not quit.

I am worth it.

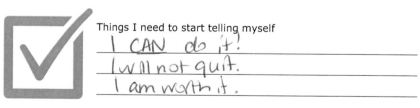

my food journal
training days

Week 1

Breakfast - Day 1	Breakfast - Day 2	Breakfast - Day 3
Lunch - Day 1	Lunch - Day 2	Lunch - Day 3
Dinner - Day 1	Dinner - Day 2	Dinner - Day 3
Water - Day 1	Water - Day 2	Water - Day 3
Other Beverages	Other Beverages	Other Beverages

my exercise journal
training days

Week 1

Day 1	Day 2	Day3
Day 1	Day 2	Day3
Day 1	Day 2	Day3

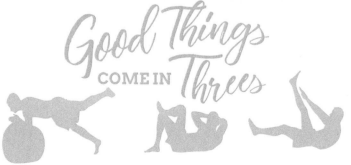

Good Things COME IN *Threes*

my recovery journal
time to recover

Week 1

Day 1	Day 2	Day3
Day 1	Day 2	Day3
Day 1	Day 2	Day3

On your rest days, take a few minutes to journal your journey! Document what you are learning about your body, how you feel, your thoughts, your fears, your progress.

...and Relax

my food journal
training days

Week 2

Breakfast - Day 1	Breakfast - Day 2	Breakfast - Day 3
Lunch - Day 1	Lunch - Day 2	Lunch - Day 3
Dinner - Day 1	Dinner - Day 2	Dinner - Day 3
Water - Day 1	Water - Day 2	Water - Day 3
Other Beverages	Other Beverages	Other Beverages

my exercise journal
training days

Week 2

Day 1	Day 2	Day3

Day 1	Day 2	Day3

Day 1	Day 2	Day3

A higher fat and fiber lifestyle, low in refined carbohydrates, plus sufficient and suitably intense exercise, will alleviate some of the worst side effects of aging.

These include, insulin resistance and increased fat mass, that will in turn greatly lower the risk of heart disease, cancer and diabetes, obesity and insulin resistance, that cause aging.

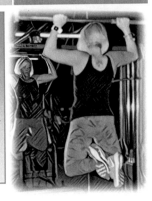

my recovery journal
time to recover

Week 2

Day 1	Day 2	Day3
Day 1	Day 2	Day3
Day 1	Day 2	Day3

On your rest days, take a few minutes to journal your journey! Document what you are learning about your body, how you feel, your thoughts, your fears, your progress.

...and Relax

my food journal
training days

Week 3

Breakfast - Day 1	Breakfast - Day 2	Breakfast - Day 3
Lunch - Day 1	Lunch - Day 2	Lunch - Day 3
Dinner - Day 1	Dinner - Day 2	Dinner - Day 3
Water - Day 1	Water - Day 2	Water - Day 3
Other Beverages	Other Beverages	Other Beverages

my exercise journal

Week 3

training days

Day 1	Day 2	Day3
Day 1	Day 2	Day3
Day 1	Day 2	Day3

"EXCUSES DON'T GET RESULTS."

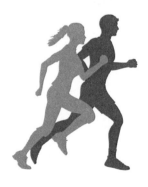

my recovery journal
time to recover

Week 3

Day 1	Day 2	Day3
Day 1	Day 2	Day3
Day 1	Day 2	Day3

On your rest days, take a few minutes to journal your journey! Document what you are learning about your body, how you feel, your thoughts, your fears, your progress.

...and
Relax

my food journal

training days

Week 4

Breakfast - Day 1	Breakfast - Day 2	Breakfast - Day 3
Lunch - Day 1	Lunch - Day 2	Lunch - Day 3
Dinner - Day 1	Dinner - Day 2	Dinner - Day 3
Water - Day 1	Water - Day 2	Water - Day 3
Other Beverages	Other Beverages	Other Beverages

my exercise journal
training days
Week 4

Day 1	Day 2	Day3
Day 1	Day 2	Day3
Day 1	Day 2	Day3

Journal it.... Use this space to document how you feel, where your mind is at... how your body feels., what your struggles are.

_____

_____

_____

_____

_____

my recovery journal

Week 4

time to recover

Day 1	Day 2	Day3

Day 1	Day 2	Day3

Day 1	Day 2	Day3

On your rest days, take a few minutes to journal your journey! Document what you are learning about your body, how you feel, your thoughts, your fears, your progress.

...and Relax

YES
YOU CAN!

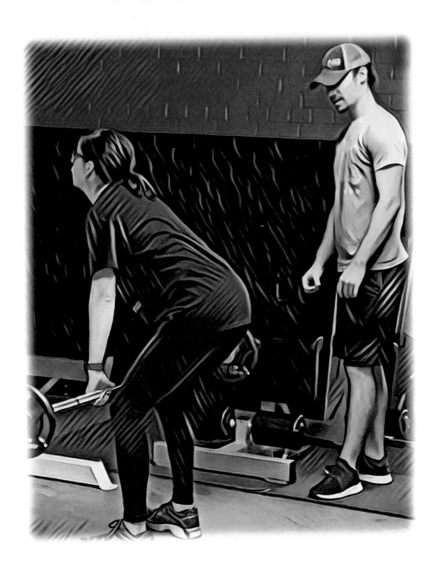

my food journal
training days

Week 5

Breakfast - Day 1	Breakfast - Day 2	Breakfast - Day 3
Lunch - Day 1	Lunch - Day 2	Lunch - Day 3
Dinner - Day 1	Dinner - Day 2	Dinner - Day 3
Water - Day 1	Water - Day 2	Water - Day 3
Other Beverages	Other Beverages	Other Beverages

my exercise journal
training days

Week 5

Day 1	Day 2	Day3
Day 1	Day 2	Day3
Day 1	Day 2	Day3

I'M GOING TO MAKE
YOU SO PROUD.
-NOTE TO SELF

my recovery journal
time to recover
Week 5

Day 1	Day 2	Day3

Day 1	Day 2	Day3

Day 1	Day 2	Day3

On your rest days, take a few minutes to journal your journey! Document what you are learning about your body, how you feel, your thoughts, your fears, your progress.

...and Relax

my food journal
training days

Week 6

Breakfast - Day 1	Breakfast - Day 2	Breakfast - Day 3
Lunch - Day 1	Lunch - Day 2	Lunch - Day 3
Dinner - Day 1	Dinner - Day 2	Dinner - Day 3
Water - Day 1	Water - Day 2	Water - Day 3
Other Beverages	Other Beverages	Other Beverages

my exercise journal
training days

Week 6

Day 1	Day 2	Day3
Day 1	Day 2	Day3
Day 1	Day 2	Day3

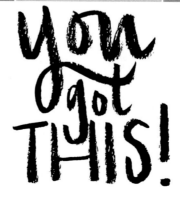

my recovery journal
time to recover

Week 6

Day 1	Day 2	Day3
Day 1	Day 2	Day3
Day 1	Day 2	Day3

On your rest days, take a few minutes to journal your journey! Document what you are learning about your body, how you feel, your thoughts, your fears, your progress.

...and Relax

my food journal
training days

Week 7

Breakfast - Day 1	Breakfast - Day 2	Breakfast - Day 3
Lunch - Day 1	Lunch - Day 2	Lunch - Day 3
Dinner - Day 1	Dinner - Day 2	Dinner - Day 3
Water - Day 1	Water - Day 2	Water - Day 3
Other Beverages	Other Beverages	Other Beverages

my exercise journal
training days

Week 7

Day 1	Day 2	Day3
Day 1	**Day 2**	**Day3**
Day 1	**Day 2**	**Day3**

IF IT DOESN'T CHALLENGE YOU, IT DOESN'T CHANGE YOU

my recovery journal
time to recover

Week 7

Day 1	Day 2	Day3
Day 1	Day 2	Day3
Day 1	Day 2	Day3

On your rest days, take a few minutes to journal your journey! Document what you are learning about your body, how you feel, your thoughts, your fears, your progress.

...and Relax

my food journal
training days

Week 8

Breakfast - Day 1	Breakfast - Day 2	Breakfast - Day 3
Lunch - Day 1	Lunch - Day 2	Lunch - Day 3
Dinner - Day 1	Dinner - Day 2	Dinner - Day 3
Water - Day 1	Water - Day 2	Water - Day 3
Other Beverages	Other Beverages	Other Beverages

my exercise journal
training days

Week 8

Day 1	Day 2	Day3
Day 1	Day 2	Day3
Day 1	Day 2	Day3

TOO TIRED
TOO BUSY
TOO WEAK

NO EXCUSES

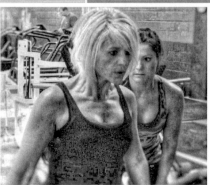

my recovery journal
time to recover

Week 8

Day 1	Day 2	Day3
Day 1	Day 2	Day3
Day 1	Day 2	Day3

On your rest days, take a few minutes to journal your journey! Document what you are learning about your body, how you feel, your thoughts, your fears, your progress.

...and
Relax

my food journal
training days

Week 9

Breakfast - Day 1	Breakfast - Day 2	Breakfast - Day 3
Lunch - Day 1	Lunch - Day 2	Lunch - Day 3
Dinner - Day 1	Dinner - Day 2	Dinner - Day 3
Water - Day 1	Water - Day 2	Water - Day 3
Other Beverages	Other Beverages	Other Beverages

my exercise journal
training days

Week 9

Day 1	Day 2	Day3
Day 1	Day 2	Day3
Day 1	Day 2	Day3

TODAY I ~~HAVE TO~~ WORKOUT
get to

my recovery journal

Week 9

time to recover

Day 1	Day 2	Day3
Day 1	Day 2	Day3
Day 1	Day 2	Day3

On your rest days, take a few minutes to journal your journey! Document what you are learning about your body, how you feel, your thoughts, your fears, your progress.

...and Relax

my food journal

training days

Week 10

Breakfast - Day 1	Breakfast - Day 2	Breakfast - Day 3
Lunch - Day 1	Lunch - Day 2	Lunch - Day 3
Dinner - Day 1	Dinner - Day 2	Dinner - Day 3
Water - Day 1	Water - Day 2	Water - Day 3
Other Beverages	Other Beverages	Other Beverages

my exercise journal
training days

Week 10

Day 1	Day 2	Day3
Day 1	Day 2	Day3
Day 1	Day 2	Day3

fearless

my recovery journal

time to recover

Week 10

Day 1	Day 2	Day3
Day 1	Day 2	Day3
Day 1	Day 2	Day3

On your rest days, take a few minutes to journal your journey! Document what you are learning about your body, your eating habits, your food addictions.

...and
Relax

my food journal
training days

Week 11

Breakfast - Day 1	Breakfast - Day 2	Breakfast - Day 3
Lunch - Day 1	Lunch - Day 2	Lunch - Day 3
Dinner - Day 1	Dinner - Day 2	Dinner - Day 3
Water - Day 1	Water - Day 2	Water - Day 3
Other Beverages	Other Beverages	Other Beverages

my exercise journal
training days

Week 11

Day 1	Day 2	Day3
Day 1	Day 2	Day3
Day 1	Day 2	Day3

Ohhh...yes ! ! !

my recovery journal
time to recover

Week 11

Day 1	Day 2	Day3
Day 1	Day 2	Day3
Day 1	Day 2	Day3

On your rest days, take a few minutes to journal your journey! Document what you are learning about your body, how you feel, your thoughts, your fears, your progress.

...and
Relax

my food journal
training days

Week 12

Breakfast - Day 1	Breakfast - Day 2	Breakfast - Day 3
Lunch - Day 1	Lunch - Day 2	Lunch - Day 3
Dinner - Day 1	Dinner - Day 2	Dinner - Day 3
Water - Day 1	Water - Day 2	Water - Day 3
Other Beverages	Other Beverages	Other Beverages

my exercise journal
training days

Week 12

Day 1	Day 2	Day3
Day 1	Day 2	Day3
Day 1	Day 2	Day3

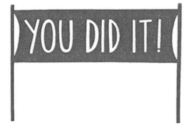

my recovery journal
time to recover

Week 12

Day 1	Day 2	Day3

Day 1	Day 2	Day3

Day 1	Day 2	Day3

On your rest days, take a few minutes to journal your journey! Document what you are learning about your body, how you feel, your thoughts, your fears, your progress.

...and Relax

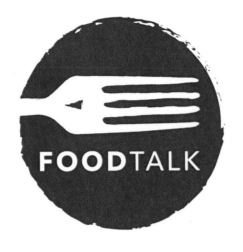

This lifestyle also involves regular physical activity, sharing meals with other people and enjoying life. Eating like a Po3 Fit Family is more of a lifestyle than a diet. Instead of gobbling your meal in front of the TV, slow down and sit down at the table with your family and friends to savor what you're eating. Not only will you enjoy your company and your food, eating slowly allows you to tune in to your body's hunger and fullness signals. You're more apt to eat until you're satisfied than until you're busting-at-the-seams full.

Here are some examples of fun fit power of 3 family meals

Breakfast Casserole with Tomatoes, Green Pepper and Goat Cheese.

This marvelous breakfast recipe combines tomatoes, green pepper and crumbled Goat cheese on top. Preparation time: 10 minutes Cooking time: 45 minutes Serves: 4-6

Ingredients:

1 green bell pepper, seeded and cut into thin strips

Olive oil, for brushing the baking pan

½ teaspoon dried oregano

1 cup cherry tomatoes, halved

¾ cup Goat cheese, crumbled

10 eggs Salt and freshly ground black pepper for seasoning the eggs

Directions:1. Preheat oven to 375 ° F (190 ° C). 2. Coat a round baking pan, including the sides, with olive oil. 3. Place the green pepper in the baking pan, sprinkle with the dried oregano and roast in the oven for 7-8 minutes. 4. In a small bowl, beat the eggs until frothy. Season with salt and black pepper. 5. Add the cherry tomatoes to the baking dish, slightly mix with the green pepper and roast in the oven for another 12-15 minutes, until the tomatoes have shriveled. 6. Top the roasted vegetables with the crumbled Goat cheese and then add the beaten eggs. 7. Place the pan back in the oven and bake for about 25 minutes, until the eggs are set and the top is golden brown. 8. Remove from the oven, slice and serve warm.

Power Breakfast with Mushrooms and Tomatoes

Reading the list of ingredients you can understand that you are about to make an absolutely delicious breakfast, which is full of vitamins and proteins. Preparation time: 5 minutes Cooking time: 15 minutes Serves: 1

Ingredients:

½ cup egg whites

3 tablespoons olive oil

½ cup thinly sliced mushrooms

½ medium tomato, thinly sliced Salt and pepper, to taste

½ cup crumbled fresh goat cheese, or cheese of your choice

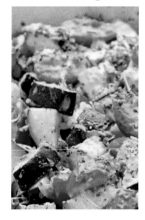

Directions: 1. Preheat the oven to 400 ° F (200 ° C). 2. Add the egg whites to a small bowl, season with salt and pepper, and beat until soft peaks have formed. 3. Add the olive oil to a large oven proof pan and set over a medium-high heat. Stir in the mushrooms and cook until tender, about 5 minutes. 4. Top the mushrooms with tomato slices. 5. Add the crumbled cheese into the egg mixture, slightly stir, and pour evenly over the tomatoes. 6. Transfer the pan to the preheated oven and bake for 7-8 minutes. 7. Remove the pan from the oven and carefully flip the dish over onto a serving plate.

Garlic Parmesan Zucchini and Tomato Bake

This recipe makes a healthy lunch which is easy to assemble as it utilizes ingredients that are always on hand. Preparation time: 5 minutes Cooking time: 30 minutes Serves: 6

Ingredients:

2 large zucchinis, cut into quarters

10oz (280g) grape tomatoes, diced

½ cup Parmesan Cheese, shredded

7 garlic cloves, crushed

1 teaspoon basil, dried

1 teaspoon thyme, dried

1 teaspoon oregano, dried

¾ teaspoon salt

½ teaspoon ground black pepper

⅓ cup parsley or basil, finely chopped Cooking spray

Directions: Preheat oven to 350 ° F (175 ° C) and coat a baking dish with cooking spray. Mix together the cheese, basil, thyme, oregano, cloves, zucchini, tomatoes, salt and pepper in a large bowl. Place the mixture into the prepared baking dish and bake in the oven for 25-30, until the vegetables are tender and the cheese is melted. Remove the bake from the oven, garnish with the chopped basil or parsley, and serve warm.

The LBB's Spicy P3 Fish Stew

comfort on a rainy day 4 serving

Ingredients

1 pound wild caught cod or other wild caught white fish- I use cod

1 pound of shrimp

1 medium lime, juiced

1 medium jalapeno pepper (seeds removed)

1 medium onion

1 medium red pepper

1 medium yellow pepper

2 cloves garlic, minced or pressed

1 teaspoon organic paprika

2 cups chicken bone-broth

2 cups chopped tomatoes

1+ teaspoons sea salt (real salt)

1/4 teaspoon Fine Ground Black Pepper

15 ounces organic coconut milk (canned)

Optional garnishes

chopped fresh cilantro

additional lime wedges

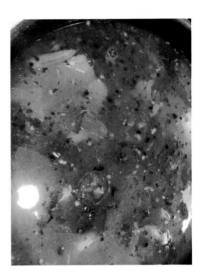

Instructions

Place the fish in a large nonreactive mixing bowl, add the lime juice, and set aside to marinate while you proceed with the recipe.

Heat a large sauté pan over medium/high heat, and add the olive oil. Once it is hot, add the peppers and onions sauté, stirring often, until the onions are translucent, 3 to 4 minutes. Add the garlic and sauté for 30 seconds.

Add the spices, tomatoes and broth, stir well to incorporate. Bring the mixture to a boil. Then add the fish (with the lime juice) and the coconut milk. Stir to combine, and bring the liquid to a boil. Cover the pan, reduce the heat to medium-low, and cook until the flesh of the fish starts to flake, about 10 minutes.

Remove the cover, sprinkle the cilantro over the fish, and serve accompanied by wedges of lime.... you can also dice a small avocado to top with as well.

Eat less sugar.
You're sweet enough already.

Baked Cod with Roasted Vegetables

Fish likes spice! Garlic, black pepper and citrus juice make this dish an unforgettable experience, which is, by the way, not difficult to achieve.

Preparation time: 20 minutes Cooking time: 45 minutes Serves: 2

Ingredients: Half a head of purple cabbage, sliced thinly
1 sweet or red onion, sliced
4 cloves garlic, chopped
1 ½ cups broccoli florets
1 green sweet pepper, sliced into strips
2 carrots, sliced into strips
⅓ cup extra virgin olive oil
¼ cup balsamic vinegar
⅓ cup apricot preserves
2 cloves garlic, minced Sea salt, to taste
Freshly ground pepper, to taste
½ teaspoon mild or hot curry
A dab of honey mustard (optional)
For the fish: 2 single cod fillets (or one large fillet, cut in half)
Extra virgin olive oil
2-3 cloves garlic, chopped
A squeeze of citrus (lemon, lime or orange)
Sea salt, to taste Freshly ground pepper, to taste

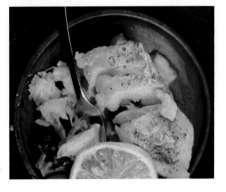

Directions: 1. Preheat the oven to 400ºF (200oC) and position the rack on the middle of the oven. 2. In a large bowl, place together the sliced cabbage, onion, chopped garlic, broccoli, carrots and pepper. 3. In a separate small bowl, combine the olive oil, vinegar, apricot preserves, minced garlic, curry, salt, pepper and honey (if using). 4. Pour the mixture over the vegetables and toss to coat. 5. Place the vegetables in the roasting pan and transfer to the oven. 6. Let the vegetables roast in the preheated oven until crisp-tender, for about 45 minutes. 7. When the vegetables are nearly done, or 10 minutes prior to full readiness, start cooking the fish. 8. Put the fillets in a baking dish, top with the garlic, and drizzle with the citrus juice and olive oil. Season with the salt and pepper. 9. Set the rack in the upper position in the oven. 10. Bake the fish until opaque through-out, for about 8-10 minutes. 11. Place the fish on a serving plate alongside the roasted vegetables. Pour any remaining roasting sauce over the top of the fish and vegetables, and serve.

"REMEMBER WHY YOU STARTED."

Chicken and Vegetable Kebabs

This is a must-try for poultry lovers. Make sure the chicken breasts are well marinated, which will add an unforgettable taste to the whole dish.

Preparation time: 40 minutes Cooking time: 10 minutes Serves: 6

Ingredients:

¼ cup fresh lemon juice

2 tablespoons freshly chopped Oregano, or

2 teaspoons dried oregano

2 tablespoons olive oil

1 ½ pounds skinless, boneless chicken breast, cut into 24 strips

18 (½ -inch-thick) slices zucchini

1 fennel bulb, cut into 12 wedges

12 garlic cloves, peeled

½ teaspoon salt ¼ teaspoon black pepper

Cooking spray

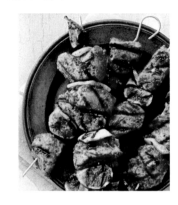

Directions: 1. Place the chicken, fennel bulb, zucchini, olive oil, lemon juice and oregano into a zip-top, heavy duty plastic bag. Seal the bag and shake well to coat. 2. Place in the refrigerator and let it marinate for 25 minutes. 3. Remove the chicken from the plastic bag and discard the marinade. 4. Prepare the grill. 5. Add the garlic cloves to a pot of boiling water and cook for 3 minutes

Remove the garlic from the water and cool. 7. Thread 3 zucchini slices, 4 chicken strips, 2 garlic cloves and 2 fennel wedges, alternately, onto the skewers and season with salt and pepper. 8. Gently coat the grill grate with cooking spray and arrange the skewers on it. 9. Grill the kebabs for about 10 minutes, until golden-brown, turning 1-2 times.

P3 Cabbage Patties

These cabbage patties will melt in your mouth. Make sure you have all the ingredients at hand and get ready for this special experience.

Preparation time: 5 minutes Cooking time: 10 minutes Serves: 2

Ingredients:

2 cups cabbage, thinly sliced

1 egg

1 green onion, chopped

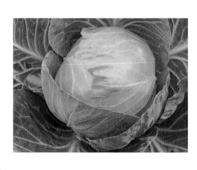

1 tablespoon olive oil , salt and pepper, to taste

Directions: 1. In a medium bowl, mix together the cabbage, onion and egg, and season with salt and pepper. 2. Add the oil to a large frying pan and set over a medium-high heat. 3. Using your hands, shape two patties from the cabbage mixture and fry in the heated pan, for about 4-5 minutes. 4. Flip over to brown the other side, then serve.

P3 Canapés with Cranberries and Goat Cheese

This is a perfect treat if you are a defender of healthy food and lifestyle, so keep this recipe safe!

Preparation time: 10 minutes Cooking time: 5 minutes Serves: 8

Ingredients: 1 teaspoon olive oil

24 walnut halves

⅛ teaspoon ground cinnamon

8oz (230g) fresh goat cheese

24 thin rounds of cucumber

½ cup cranberries, dried

1 teaspoon fresh thyme, chopped

coarse salt, ground pepper

Directions: 1. Preheat oven to 375ºF (190ºC). 2. Place the walnuts on a baking tray, drizzle with 1 teaspoon oil, and sprinkle with salt, pepper and cinnamon. 3. Bake in the oven until light brown and fragrant, for about 5 minutes. Remove from the oven and let it cool. 4. Arrange the cucumber slices on a serving plate and season with salt and pepper. 5. In a medium bowl, combine the cheese and 2 tablespoons of water. 6. Toss in the cranberries, stir, and then add the thyme, salt and pepper. 7. Spread the goat cheese mixture onto the cucumber slices, garnish with walnuts and enjoy.

Flavorful Meatballs

Total Time: 45 minutes / Serves: 6

Ingredients: 2 lbs ground beef

1/ 4 tsp onion powder

1/ 2 tsp garlic powder

1/ 4 cup feta cheese, crumbled

2 tbsp parsley, chopped

2 tbsp scallions, chopped

1/ 4 cup bell pepper, roasted and chopped

1/ 4 cup olives, chopped

1/ 4 cup sun-dried tomatoes, chopped

1/ 2 tsp black pepper 1/ 2 tsp salt

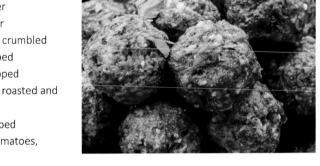

Directions: Preheat the oven to 400 F/ 204 C. Spray a baking tray with cooking spray and set aside. In a large mixing bowl, combine together all ingredients. Make small meatballs from mixture and place on a baking tray. Bake in preheated oven for 15 minutes then flip meatballs and cook for another 10 minutes. Serve and enjoy.

Power of 3 Baked Salmon

Salmon topped with healthy vegetables tastes fantastic. Check out this preparation method and see that it is as good as promised.

Preparation time: 5 minutes Cooking time: 22 minutes Serves: 4

Ingredients:

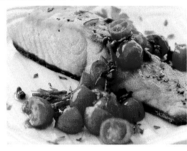

4 (6oz/ 170g) salmon fillets, skinless

2 cups cherry tomatoes, halved

½ cup zucchini, finely chopped

2 tablespoons capers, un-drained

1 tablespoon olive oil

1 (2.25oz/ 60g) can sliced ripe olives, drained

¼ teaspoon salt

¼ teaspoon black pepper

Cooking spray

Directions; 1. Preheat the oven to 425oF (220o C). 2. Season the fish with the salt and pepper on both sides. 3. Gently oil a baking dish with the cooking spray and arrange the fish fillets on the tray. 4. In a bowl, combine the cherry tomatoes, zucchini, capers and olive oil. Stir to mix well before pouring this mixture over the fish. 5. Bake in the oven for 20-22 minutes, or until the fish is cooked through.

STOP LETTING FOOD BE THE BOSS OF YOU

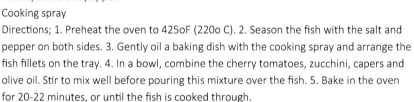

you're gonna need this
STUFF

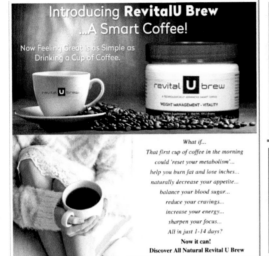

Introducing **RevitalU Brew**
...A Smart Coffee!

Now Feeling Great is as Simple as Drinking a Cup of Coffee.

revital **U** brew

WEIGHT MANAGEMENT - VITALITY

What if...
That first cup of coffee in the morning
could 'reset your metabolism'...
help you burn fat and lose inches...
naturally decrease your appetite...
balance your blood sugar...
reduce your cravings...
increase your energy...
sharpen your focus...
All in just 1-14 days?
Now it can!
Discover All Natural Revital U Brew

To join the Po3 Facebook
page for recipes,
exercise routines,
LIVE FEEDS and more,
use the code below.

PO3book1

BULLETPROOF COFFEE

1 CUP OF COFFEE

2 TBSP KERRY GOLD BUTTER

1 TBSP COCONUT OIL

www.revitalu.com/jena

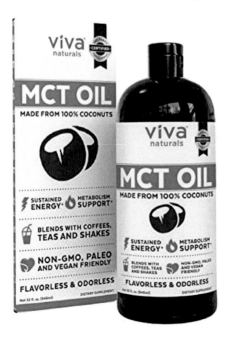

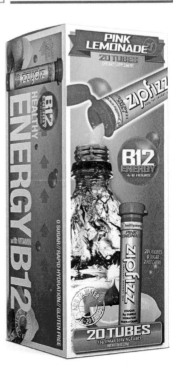

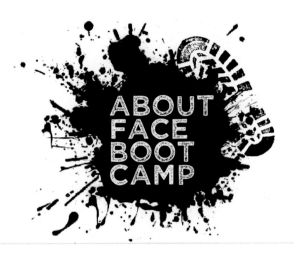

8 WEEK FIT CHALLENGE

Do you need to LOSE 50lbs, 75lbs, or 100LBS or MORE?

THIS PROGRAM INCLUDES:

- 3 CLASSES A WEEK
- MEAL PLAN
- ACCOUNTABILITY
- PRIVATE FACEBOOK GROUP

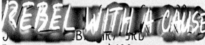

THIS PROGRAM IS $100

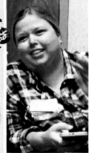
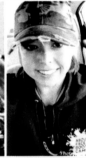
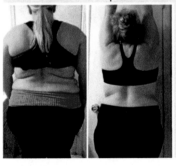
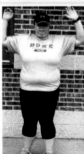
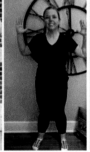

117 Center Street Cramerton, NC 28032 704-879-4105

YOU DID IT! You have completed 12 weeks of the best decision you have ever made. Your body has changed, your mind has changed, your eating habits have changed...
JUST LOOK AT YOU!

I encourage you to continue your journey. Don't go back, you've come way to far. If you haven't already, grab a friend and take them with you. An accountability partner makes all the difference and now that you've been through this transformation, you're the perfect person to lead the way for someone else.

Changing the way you eat, exercising your body and resetting your mind is not about being a size 2, being a hot mom, or even being sexy. Its about preserving your life. Preventing yourself from cardiovascular disease, diabetes, depression, strokes and even cancer.

Congratulations on this great achievement! The best is yet to come!
Now take a selfie and show off a little :)

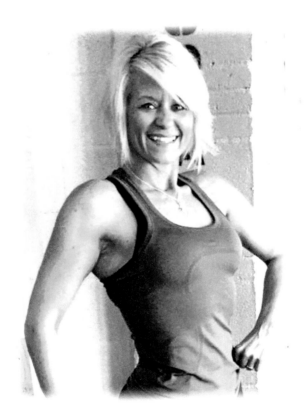

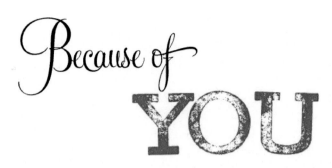

I dedicate this book to those of you who have spent your entire life following all the dieting "rules" ....only to feel like a failure. It's time to Reject the Diet Culture - it's done a number on us! The Power of 3 helps begin to undo the damage by developing the skills to call out diet BS when you see it and get MAD AS HECK about the lies we've been sold. It forces you to recognize that weight loss & the diet mentality is doing more harm than good and helps you ditch the tools that keep you chained to diet culture - whether it's your Women's Health subscription, your calorie tracker app, or just your scales.

With a heart filled with Gratitude...I would like to thank my beautiful daughter, Amie, who has taught me that having the courage to love makes you stronger...

To my bonus sons, Jake and Zack... Thank you for teaching me to love without Borders...

To The love of my life..., Gary... thank you for teaching me that you can find the perfect love you even while you're not perfect...

To my Bestie... Misty, thank you for loving me at my worst and encouraging me to become my best ....

And to Deborah Ray ... thank you for turning my words into a beautiful masterpiece, for your hard work and dedication and helping me complete this God ordained project... I love you my Bonita!

Jena ♡

Jennifer H. Armstrong

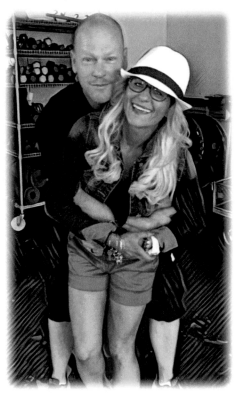

- AKA "the little blonde beast"
- Age: 45
- A mother of 3; one daughter and two "bonus boys" and living happily ever after with her fiancé in North Carolina
- Occupation: Gym Owner Contest Prep and Transformation Specialist
- Experience: 18 years
- Credentials: Certified Personal Trainer, Sports Nutrition Specialist
- Author of , "Hey Girl Hey, & ModesTea , both available on Amazon

- Certified Physique & Figure Training Specialist, NPC Bikini Competitor, NPC Fitness Competitor, Run Coach, Bodybuilding Pro Card with the ANBF, Ultra Marathon Runner
- Polar Ambassador
- Sponsored Athlete of Nutrishop
- Motivational Life Coach

My Mission in Life
I want to change the way you see your body &
show you how strong you are!
To show you that there are no limits - except for the ones
you create in your own minds by fear ....

~ Jena

Made in the USA
San Bernardino, CA
25 July 2018